The
5-Minute
Mindset
for Weight Loss

Bob Hoffman

Published 2011 by Bob Hoffman, Sandy, Utah

Library of Congress Catalog Card #: 2011902619

ISBN: 978-0-9832412-0-1

Visit us at: www.The5-MinuteMindset.com

Table of Contents

Introduction

When I finally decided that weight loss was a priority in my life I changed my mindset so powerfully that I took action and lost 73 pounds in five months.

This book is about developing the right mindset for weight loss.

In the past I tried losing weight and like many of you I lost some, and then put it right back on plus some extra pounds. Then I would try something else with the same result. I tried the advice of doctors, nutritionists and friends; I failed again and again. Why? I didn't have the right mindset.

Not until I developed the right mindset was I able to change my eating and exercise habits and keep the weight off, all 73 pounds; almost three twenty five pound bags of sugar.

After I lost all that weight, people began asking me how I did it. I told them it was a combination of things; I changed my eating and exercise habits and had the right mindset.

Many people didn't understand what I meant by 'the right mindset.'

The dictionary defines mindset as the mental attitude, inclination, or habit that you use when approaching a situation, especially one that may be perceived as being difficult or challenging.

But how do you develop the right mindset?

As friends and family continued to ask me about what I had done, I came up with nine specific steps that I used to create the right mindset for weight loss.

As you read this book you will learn the steps for developing a successful mindset and how to use them. I call this system, **The 5-Minute Mindset for Weight Loss.**

Each step is overviewed and examples provided of how to implement each step. As you learn the steps and engage in this process, you'll be firmly on the path to a healthier and happier lifestyle.

The 5-Minute Mindset for Weight Loss is about developing the right mindset needed to change eating and exercise habits permanently. Once in place, it only takes about five minutes a day to maintain.

Remembering and using these powerful principles, strengthens your resolve and shortens the time it takes to form new habits and change your life in meaningful and significant ways. It is one of the easiest and most reliable systems for weight loss even if you hate dieting and exercise.

Apply what you learn from **The 5-Minute Mindset for Weight Loss** and enjoy your success as you achieve your weight loss goals.

Step 1
Decide Now to Lose Weight

Do you really want to lose weight? Until you decide that weight loss is a priority, you will make little or no progress. Do you have the desire to lose weight? How strong is your desire? How can you increase your desire?

Our actions show what our real desires are. For example: You say you want to lose weight but you continue to eat French fries and drink soft drinks. You choose to ignore how the fat grams and calories in these foods affect your weight.

When you decide you want to lose weight and are serious about it, your actions change and you begin developing the right mindset.

While this first step sounds simple, it is one of the keys to your success. Before you can change the habits that make you overweight, you have to recognize the fact that you are overweight and decide to lose those excess pounds.

Many of us continue to tell ourselves that we really aren't that overweight. There were times after purchasing a suit that I would look at myself in the mirror and think, wow I look good. In fact I was about 130 pounds over weight and purchasing the largest suit in the store. Only my mother thought I looked good in that suit. Thanks mom.

How can you begin to lose weight until you acknowledge that you are overweight and make the decision to do something about it?

As you read this book and apply the principles, you will change the way you think about weight loss and develop the right mindset.

As I contemplated my own life, it was easy to choose weight loss as a priority. I am working on other areas of my life as well, but losing weight became a priority for a number of reasons. I fought being overweight for a long time. I tried different diets, different exercise programs, nothing seemed to work. Sound familiar?

Finally, in the process of developing the **5-Minute Mindset** system, I lost 73 pounds. I learned the difference between actually losing weight, and just dreaming about it. There were peaks and valleys in my journey but deciding to lose weight was the first step.

I suggest that you purchase our **5-Minute Mindset for Success** workbook as part of your weight loss program. Write down your current weight, take some pictures, and make the decision to lose weight now!!

Step 2
Write Your Own Story and Find Your 'Whys'

Now that you have decided losing weight is a priority in your life, it's time to write your own story. Writing your own story is about finding your 'whys'-- the reasons you want to lose weight!! Writing your own story means finding experiences from your own life which will inspire you to lose weight and writing them down. Be realistic about who you are and what you want to change. Write about whatever will motivate you to lose weight, either positive or negative.

My story took a period of time to write. I looked at experiences in my life that were occurring and wrote about them and how losing weight would improve my life. You may choose to do the same or simply make a list of reasons why you want to lose weight. For example, here is a list my sister-in-law made:

I'll fit better in my clothes.
I'll be able to go up and down stairs easier.

I'll spend less money on clothes.
I'll save money on food.
I'll enjoy looking in the mirror.

Her list continues to grow as she loses weight and realizes how it affects other areas of her life.

Finding your 'whys' can be as simple as making a list or as fun as writing about some of your life experiences like I did.

Finding your 'whys' and writing your own story may mean answering some of the following questions and putting them in writing: Why do you want to lose weight? How will losing weight improve your life? How will losing those excess pounds improve your relationships? Will your self esteem improve? How will you become more active? What will improve in your life as you lose your weight? Write down whatever will motivate and encourage you to stay on your weight loss journey. Remember, this can be in list form or in story form.

As I gained an understanding of my 'whys,' my writing began to take on a new power and focus. In particular, it helped me remember the reasons I wanted to lose weight. When I was tempted to stray from my goals, I re-read my story to regain focus.

Every day the decisions you make, what you think about, and what you do, build your life and destiny. As I began writing my own weight loss story, I realized it would take some time to achieve my weight loss goals. In the process of developing the proper mindset, it was important for me to accept myself as I was. You will find the same to be important for you.

As I began to brainstorm and think about all the reasons I did not want to be overweight, I wrote these down in some detail. As I went through this process, the commitment to develop a weight loss plan became an absolute commitment. My desire to lose weight and live healthier became so strong that I began to overcome the habits that kept me from losing weight.

As you move forward with the other steps, refer to this step and your own story for motivation. Continue adding to your story as you go through the **5-Minute Mindset** process. Writing my own story helped me remember why I wanted to lose weight and stay the course when I felt like giving up or got discouraged. Writing your own story or making a list of 'whys' strengthens your emotional attachment to your goals.

This part of the mindsetting process was so important to me that I spent a great deal of time in this area preparing for my weight loss program.

Losing 73 pounds in five months took a powerful mindset and writing my own story was a key component of that success. I also found that using creativity in writing the story such as cartoons, pictures, etc. helped me more vividly express my weight loss concerns and enhance my desire for weight loss.

The following are examples of my own stories. They are straight forward, fun and helped me develop the right mindset for my weight loss program.

Big Fat and Proud of That?
My Story

When I first began writing my story I was 130 pounds overweight. These stories are my stories and became my reasons for losing weight. Frankly, I became sick of being fat and I was certainly not 'fat and proud of that.' I was hanging on to being fat so tightly, it appeared that I was indeed proud of that.

For the rest of this section, I will share some insights about my own personal story and why I decided to change the 'proud of that' fat attitude. I hope that my stories inspire you to write your own story and change your mindset.

As I make fun of myself in the stories and pictures, many of you will relate. Don't feel bad, it may trigger ideas for your 'whys.' You will soon be on the road to a healthier, happier you.

We recognize there are medical conditions and circumstances that make losing weight very difficult, if not impossible for some. That's OK; you may find inspiration for other areas of your life that you can control and change. At the very least, you may be motivated to develop better habits.

One of the beginning steps to making a change in our lives is both accepting and loving ourselves as we are. Yes, fat and all! (Some of us have more to love than others. Aren't we lucky?)

Everyone has different skills and talents. Know that you are an amazing person. Love yourself now, be happy now, live life to its fullest now. At the same time, beginning to make some positive changes in your life will only add to your happiness. Happiness is, after all, a journey not a destination. It really isn't arriving that suddenly makes life worthwhile; it's the daily striving that makes it fun and meaningful.

I hope you find my stories helpful and in some small way, assist you in your quest to become less fat and proud of that.

Enjoy the stories and pictures, and begin writing your own story or list of 'whys' as ideas come to you.

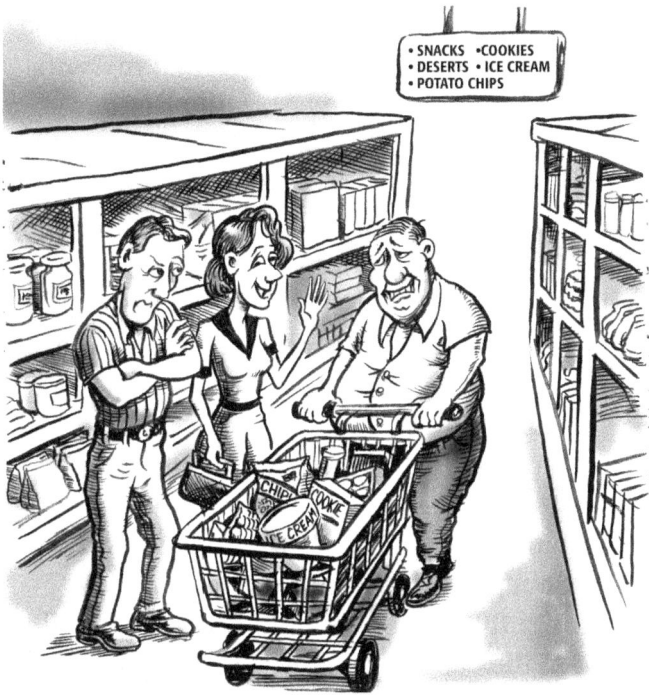

Shopping for Food

Although my wife does most of the grocery shopping, she would occasionally call me to stop and pick up a few items. A quick call while I am out and about and I'm ready to make a quick stop to pick up a couple of items for the family. If I only need to pick up a couple of items, why do I always grab the cart instead of the smaller basket? I'll tell you why. You can fill a large cart with more healthy, wonderful food like potato chips, ice cream, pop, etc.

Heaven forbid that I should actually go into the store and buy the couple of items that my wife needs to fix dinner. No way, while I'm here I'll load up.

So, here's how it went; bag of chips, chip dip, tortilla chips, cookies, ice cream, Cool Whip, an apple, (hey, who put that fruit in my basket?). OK, that does it. All I really needed was the apple and the Cool Whip. But while I'm here, let's check out the candy aisle. Yeah, get a little something for the kids, (which I do), then a couple of extra candy bars for me; one to eat on the way home, the other to eat upon arrival. And of course, there is always the exciting possibility that either the kids or my wife will not want the candy. Who was I trying to kid? I really can't understand how I got so fat? (Yeah right!!!) Personally, I got fat eating like a pig. That's it, pure, plain and simple. My motto after I return home: Start eating, and don't quit until bedtime. I could make up excuses for overeating with the best of them. Yes, there are some people who for medical or genetic reasons can't help gaining weight, but for the vast majority of us, we just eat more than we need to.

Anyway, I now have a cart full of healthy food, right? So as I wheel my cart around and prepare to check out, it dawns on me that almost everything in my cart is not exactly what would be classified as health food. I'm beginning to feel a bit guilty about it when suddenly someone called out my name. Great. Here I am with this boatload of junk food and one small apple for my wife. Where can I hide? Can I pretend not to hear them? Should I turn my cart around, and run up the aisle the other way, explaining to them later that I didn't hear them? I had seconds to decide. Then it happened, we made eye contact. All plausible excuses are now shot to pieces. So I waddled toward them. The cart seemed to weigh two tons. We exchanged greetings.

"How are things going?" they asked.

We make small talk for a minute then of course they eventually do the 'check out what the fat man bought' thing. I watched their eyes wandering over my boatload of wonderful food and I could see this look come into their eyes. I could almost read their minds, "Overdoing it just a bit aren't we? Feeding some kids in the neighborhood? Snacking for four are we?"

Oh, they were polite enough, but that look. You know it; you've seen it. I wonder what they would have thought if they had known that the snacks in the cart would be gone in one night. But, oh what a night it would be!!!

Let's further illustrate the point about the cart. Now let's assume for a minute, that the neighbors who looked in my cart don't really care what I have in it. Let's assume that no one cares what's in it. The fact is, I do. I am self conscious about what is in my shopping cart because I am so doggone fat—that's the problem.

I can't begin to tell you how many times I've told others how good my self esteem is. I really believe that it is. Nevertheless, being the butt end of jokes, comments and snide remarks does in fact get old.

The cart story doesn't end here. In fact, it reinforces how pathetic I felt to be fat and to even have to worry about any of this. So, now I finished my conversation with the neighbor and I'm pushing my cart towards the checkout stand. So, who will the checker be, the one least likely to say something about my precious junk food? Most checkers won't say anything, being highly trained in the art of not offending the fat people. After all, we do buy one heck of a lot of food. We keep those checkers busy now, don't we? So I pick out the checker that I don't think will say anything.

On this particular day, I have done very well for myself; lots of good things to eat. So, I empty the cart onto the little conveyor belt (now this is very revealing): one small apple, cookies, candy bars, potato chips, bags of candy, pop, gum, chocolate milk, and my favorite, two cartons of mint chocolate chip ice cream.

The checker is very pleasant and begins to check me out. "Wow," she says, "Looks like someone's having a party."

You bet, I say to myself, and what a party I'm going to have. I'll eat most of this junk food by myself. Certainly, my family will get a piece or two, but guess who gets to polish most of it off? Oh, yeah!! I'm the one in desperate need of a party and the party food after all.

At the time, shopping, to say the very least, was not fun. I felt extra self conscious and wished I could make the commitment to start doing something about my weight and controlling what I bought at the store.

When I picked up the snacks for the family, I sometimes asked myself the question. "When will I care enough to actually do something about this?" Of course we all know the answer to that question now don't we. We are going to start doing something about it on Monday. I planned to start losing weight every Monday for twenty years. Or, I planned to get started after the upcoming birthday party, the big celebration dinner, the vacation, Christmas, New Years, etc. We all know the story. We are going to start tomorrow and we are going to do something about it, later; certainly not today. Maybe I'll get on a weight loss plan after Thanksgiving. Have you ever done that? Thanksgiving is coming up. One last splurge, then I'm done eating like a pig, forever; Yeah, right!

Now, let's check out what really happened after Thanksgiving that year. Thanksgiving was great! Lots of family, plenty of good food to eat; Boy, it was fun! Of course, as I mentioned, maybe I'll start losing weight right after Thanksgiving. Naturally, that isn't going to work because on Friday the family goes shopping at a shopping center uptown. Now here's my rationale. I can't start losing weight on Friday because while we're shopping we have to eat someplace. So lunch is good, I love hot dogs and lemonade. Only 4,500 calories or so, but it's tasty. I'm sure that I can start eating right on Saturday.

Oops, the family is invited to eat a post Thanksgiving dinner of leftovers. Awesome!! So Saturday is out. Then Sunday rolls around and the weekend is almost over. A fantastic

Sunday dinner awaits. I am certainly not going
to start my weight loss program on Sunday.
No, I'll wait for my favorite day to begin losing
weight; Monday. So on Sunday I ate all my
regular healthy food: cookies, ice cream,
popcorn, pop, etc. Now, I know how pathetic I
sound, but I also know human nature and many
of you are procrastinating the same way.

I hope my candor in writing about some of
these issues helps you be more honest with
yourself. Recognizing you are overweight is an
important step in heading down the path to
losing weight.

You know what I'm talking about. We look in
the mirror and tell ourselves that we are not that
fat or don't even think about it. Wow, I love
my mirror. I love the self perception that I have
about the guy that shows up in the mirror. Not
too bad. I've seen worse. Yeah right, maybe at
a sumo wrestling match. Admitting that I was
overweight was an important step for me to
take.

Next, I go shopping for clothes. This is so
exciting!

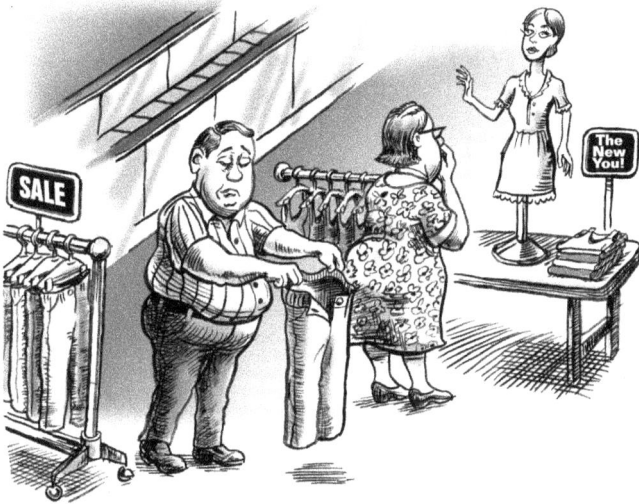

Shopping for Clothes

Here's something I really hated about being fat; shopping for clothes.

Now this is an activity that really makes us feel good about ourselves! You are forced to shop now and then because your clothes shrank, and they no longer fit, right? Many of us have hanging in our closets a few different sizes of clothes.

Personally, I have three different sizes of clothes; one size that works when I am on a regular diet and doing fairly well; one size even smaller when I am changing my eating habits and exercising and my largest size that usually gets pretty snug before I get going on some type of diet to start losing weight again. I also have suits in different sizes and to my credit I have held on to my larger clothes (doing this has saved lots of money). You know what I mean, don't you. By the way, I seem to spend most of my time in the larger size and usually they are fairly tight. Fortunately, this has changed for me and it can change for you as well.

My family would watch television and on comes the infamous "big and tall commercial." You know the store that sells clothing basically the same size as tents. I know the kids didn't mean to hurt my feelings but they kind of snickered when this commercial would come on. I wonder who they were thinking about when they saw that commercial; one of their skinny friends? Don't think so.

I was barely avoiding the big and tall stores. Frankly speaking, I knocked on the door more than once. At the time I began writing my own story I had to buy the largest waist size of pants that you could find in the department stores. If I didn't begin losing weight, I was going to be off to the tent store on my next trip. Most of us who head to that store probably aren't heading there because of our height. Personally I can't stand shopping at a grocery store let alone a clothing store for fat people. Why not call it what it is, not a Big and Tall store, but the Fatty Fatty Store or the Fat and Fatter Store? Maybe if the Big and Tall stores were properly named it would encourage more of us to work harder and avoid having to shop there.

Many times while shopping I noticed that most stores with the latest and greatest clothes didn't have them in my size. It would tick me off that they didn't carry my pant and shirt size but it is in fact the case.

Instead of being ticked off, I decided to do the smart thing and lose weight. If I were at my ideal weight, all the stores would carry my size. Fortunately for me, there were a few stores that did carry my giant pants. Maybe my wife would really have gotten after me with a vengeance if she had to sew and make clothes for me.

Shopping for clothes has never been fun for me. I disliked any type of shopping but shopping for clothes became a real pain. No matter what clothes I bought, I knew that underneath it all was still the fatty, fatty two by four; me.

I do believe that it is important to buy clothes that fit well no matter what the size.

Please believe me when I tell you that I know what it is like to be fat. What doesn't make sense to me is that as negative of a thing as it is to be fat, why didn't I do something about it?

If you relate to what I am saying I hope that my directness doesn't offend you. If it does, I'm sorry. I'm only this frank because I was writing to myself and it takes a lot to get me off the dime and take action.

Ok, back to the 'shopping for clothes' story. The last time that I bought a suit, I kid you not, I think I bought the largest size that they had available in the regular store. Man, I was so close to going to the fat store. You would think this would wake me up.

When I bought my last fatty suit, the salesperson put me in front of the mirror to make adjustments and I thought I looked good in that suit. But not all mirrors can lie. In some of the mirrors, I actually do look a little extra plump. Based on the fact that I'm wearing the biggest size available at the 'normal' store was just a little bit scary to me. Clearly the guy in the mirror with a round jolly face like mine must be one fat son of a gun.

Most clothes that are really 'in' don't come in tent sizes. While there are many stores that do cater to fat folks, face it, who really wants to shop there. I don't.

By doing something about being overweight, I'll be able to find a greater variety of clothes to wear that will be less expensive. And best of all when I look in the mirror I'll feel a lot better about myself.

Shopping is absolutely no fun, but it could be, and will be, when I lose those excess pounds permanently.

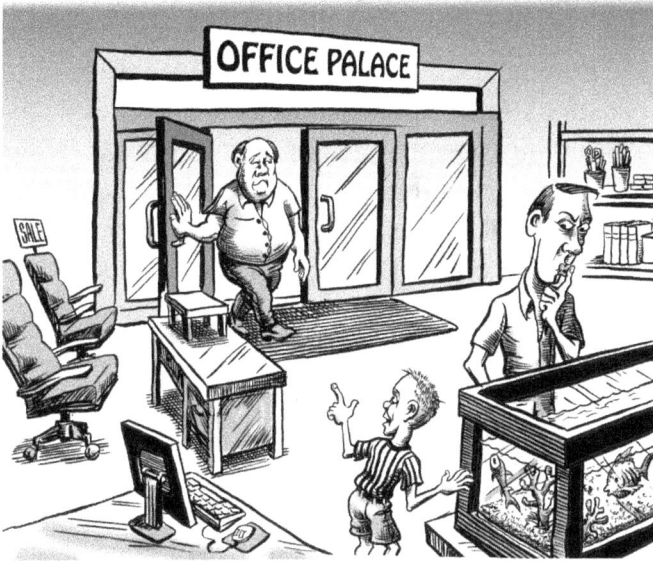

Scaring the Children

I was in the process of setting up my real estate office in a location not too far from our home. I was shopping at an office furniture store for some chairs for our reception area.

As I walked in the front door, on the right hand side was a large aquarium filled with water and a number of colorful fish. Standing in front of the aquarium was a young boy, probably three or four years old. His father was standing near by and I would guess that he was in his late 20's or early 30's. After seeing them, I turned away and walked toward the showroom where the chairs were. The showroom was quiet and there was no one else in the area. Suddenly, I heard this small voice boom out this question. "Daddy, how do people get a fat tummy?" Now let's think about this. What caused this sudden interest in fat tummies? Hmm; was he referring to me? Since only three people were in the showroom, a small boy, a skinny dad, and me, who was he asking about?

So as I looked at the furniture, I continued listening to the conversation that ensued between the boy and his dad. This would be interesting. The dad knows I'm within easy earshot and his boy is talking very loud. How would he handle this? Without skipping a beat, the dad replied to his son's question, "Because God made them that way." Not a bad answer for someone put on the spot. The young father should have been given an award for being tactful. Really, what else could he say? "Well, that man is probably fat because he eats like a pig, and he'll probably die at 50 because his heart will quit beating, and he's responsible for our health and life insurance premiums being so high." Or, "He's fat because he consumes so many fat grams he needs a calculator to add them up every day." To his credit he handled the matter very tactfully.

His son's next question was also very interesting. "Dad, are fat people mean?" Well of course we are. At that point I should have run (or waddled) back up the aisle as fast as I could, screaming at the top of my lungs, baring my fangs, looking like the giant Stay Puff marshmallow boy in Ghostbusters and given the boy a good scare. But being the mature person that I am, I just tuned in to hear what the dad would say. Again the dad gave a respectable answer. "No, fat people aren't mean, they're nice just like normal people."

After the dad said that, I wasn't too sure what to think about his answer. Do fat people have some different classification in life? Was I something other than normal? What exactly would that be? That was all I heard at that point as I walked up the hall a little faster and yes, a little more contemplative.

What a sad state of affairs. My being overweight had caused a young father a couple of uncomfortable moments. The big question in my mind was, did this little boy express what everyone is actually thinking when they see a fat person but are too polite to speak their minds? I knew that this young boy was just being straightforward with his thoughts and wasn't in any way trying to be mean, but had I allowed myself to become so heavy that I had a

different classification other than 'normal?'
Anyway I certainly found it interesting that fat
people could be nice just like 'normal' people.
So maybe being at a lower weight makes you
more normal? So you see, shopping can be a
real neat experience when you're fat, no matter
where we go and what we shop for.

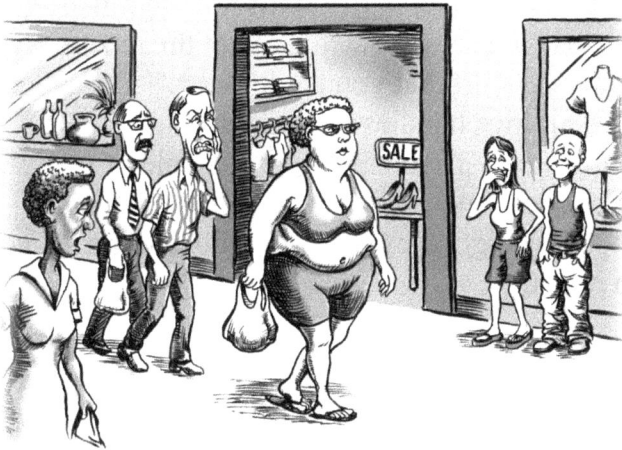

Spandex Can Be Terrifying

There are, without question a number of things
that heavy folks shouldn't do. Wearing tight
fitting spandex is definitely one of these things.
Give me a break. I was in the mall once when
this huge overweight gal comes walking down
the hall wearing tight fitting spandex. Believe
thee me, it was scary. OK; if you are
overweight, for crying out loud, do your best
not to accentuate the fact that you're 150
pounds overweight. Besides, scaring the public
like that might cause accidents and land you in
jail.

My wife reminds me from time to time not to wear the pullover shirts that I love so much because in her words, "that's not the most flattering shirt that you could wear." Let's face it; giant love handles really aren't that attractive. I personally have a couple of pretty good sized ones. I've decided that after I lose enough weight, then I'll wear those shirts I love so much.

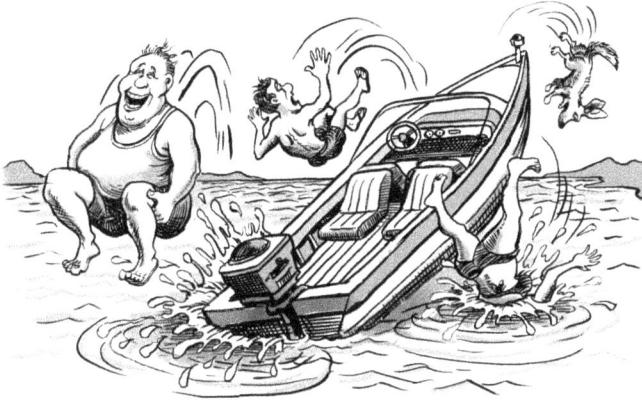

Boating as a Fat Man

A number of years ago our family decided to take up boating; a wholesome, healthy activity our family could do together. They love knee boarding, tubing, swimming, and enjoy the lakes and being outdoors. We've had many experiences that we can remember and laugh about years later. So far, after 17 years of boating, almost all of our experiences have been fun. It has been and continues to be an activity the whole family still loves to do.

So is boating as fun for a person who is overweight? I follow my wife's advice about what to wear. When we go boating I wear my size 50 XXXL swimming suit. Gratefully, they make swimming suits in my size, although usually the choices are limited and many times not that attractive. I also wear a large t-shirt to protect both the public from an eyesore of an extra 100 pounds of blubber and myself from sunburn. (As a fat guy, I have so much more to burn.)

So life is good, everyone is happy until it's time to get in the water. Face it. You will either get in to ski, swim or whatever, but you aren't going to own a boat and not get into the water. So, here comes the scary part. My family enjoys a particular part of the lake that we affectionately call the 'swimming hole.' It's a small cove like area where no skiing is allowed. Here the kids love to anchor the boat, eat, swim, sun bathe, etc. Usually they swim and use the boat as a diving board. They do have a blast.

So here we are at the swimming hole. On a hot day you just have to get into the water. Suddenly there's a huge white flash. You think that it's some type of a huge light explosion. Actually, it's just me taking off my t-shirt so I can put on a life jacket. Believe me, I light up the whole area. One of the advantages of the brightness created by my white skin, is everyone is temporarily blinded so I can hurry and put on my life jacket and get into the water. Actually, I will normally jump off the back of the boat, cannon ball style, creating somewhat of a huge tidal wave. The boat rocks, the kids bob up and down in the tsunami, and everyone knows that dad has just entered the water. Thankfully, the kids like the wave and don't normally make fun of me.

My family has always been great about my overweight problem; they don't tease me about my weight, most of the time. They are awesome and totally accepting of me. I love and appreciate them for that. Taking off my t-shirt and revealing my giant love handles and rolls of fat has been very embarrassing for me. I participated in all the family activities but I began asking myself the question, "Hey fatty; when are you going to do something about this weight?" Wouldn't it be nice if I could take that shirt off and not be embarrassed about it? Let's face it; being fat really hasn't been all that beautiful.

Even if you're fat, I personally believe it's important to participate as much as you can in your family's traditions and activities, and enjoy them to the best of your ability. Being fat detracts from your quality of life. That's the reality. By losing that excess weight you can live a fuller, happier life and enjoy your family activities and traditions more.

One week we were at our favorite swimming hole while we were boating. The girls had brought friends and one of them just happened to be a guy; tall, slender, in great shape. He could dive off the end of the boat, doing back flips, forward flips; he was amazing. All of their friends seemed very nice. So, when I got into the water, after scaring everyone by taking off my shirt, it was nice to just stay in the water for a while. It was especially nice for me because no one could see my love handles through the water.

Now comes the hard part; getting back onto the boat. Hard for a couple of reasons; one, I didn't want my kids' friends to see me fighting my way back onto the boat with my whale like body; and two, I have to be careful not to break the ladder. I'm sure that my weight on the ladder was not a good thing. So, I try to support myself with my arms to minimize the weight on the ladder. But isn't it sad I even have to think this way? Wouldn't it be nice to be less fat and therefore less self conscious about things? Admit it. You know that I am right; you get tired of being heavy as well.

Boating and other outdoor activities would be a lot more fun if you're not overweight.

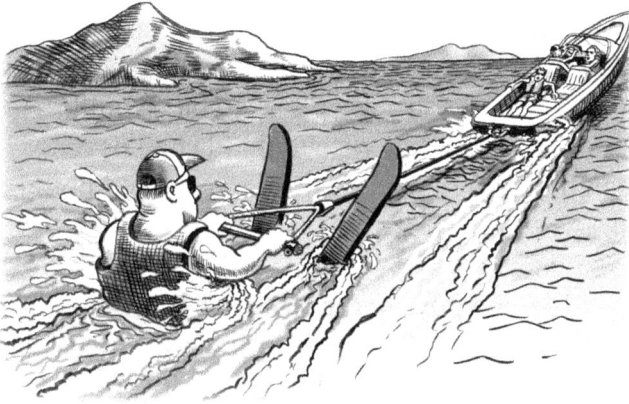

My Saddest Boating Day Ever

Let me share one more boating experience. As a young man about the age of 14, I went water skiing for the first time at a wonderful lake called Lake Powell. I can remember laying there in the water, yelling at Bruce, the driver, to hit it, and up I came. Yep. First time up, and away I went. I certainly thought that I was a hot shot to be able to get up and ski my very first try.

Now, years later, getting up to ski has become increasingly difficult. However, even with the added weight, I have always been able to get up and do a little skiing. Sometimes it has taken a try or two to get up, but hey, what do you expect with a little extra weight and a few extra

years? However, for a person with an ego the
size of mine, the unthinkable in fact happened; I
could not get up. As impossible as it seemed,
disaster finally struck. I was so fat I couldn't
get up and ski. My wife and kids had never
seen this before. But, true story, I could not get
up.

I felt like the guy on the commercial where the
big fat guy is in the water with his skis and he is
telling the driver of the boat to hit it. But the
driver has already 'hit it,' in fact, the driver is
flooring it and the boat does not move. The guy
is too heavy for the boat to pull him. In my
case, the boat did move but I could not get up.
It is so lovely to be fat. Isn't it great?

Time to do something about it, isn't it?

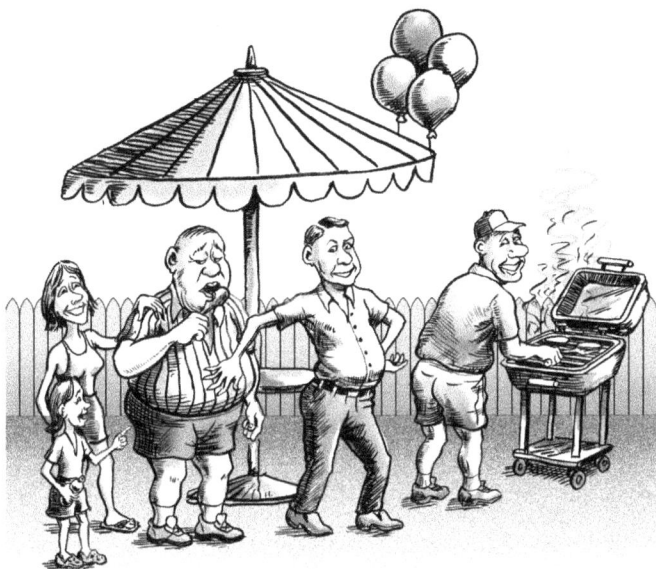

You'll Enjoy Yourself More at Social and Family Functions

Families are great. I married into a family that really has their organizational acts together with respect to family traditions. My wife's family had had many activities over the years. They organize summer time reunions and celebrate Thanksgiving, Christmas, Mother's Day, Father's Day, birthdays, etc. My family has been participating in these activities for over 31 years; it's been great. My kids have grown up knowing who their cousins are; not just their names, but actually playing with them when they were younger. Our extended family is great together and we really enjoy our time with them.

When I was first married, I was a little reluctant to go to the activities but soon warmed up to the idea and have enjoyed being around such wonderful people for many years. Over the years as I became overweight, a few family members made it their duty to make fun of my weight. Being fat is hard enough. Being made fun of by others, especially family, isn't fun at all.

In our family I have a niece that married a fine young man. He is a hard worker and a really good guy. But for some reason he believes it's his responsibility to remind me of just how fat I am.

"Hey there Uncle Bob, you're looking just a little bit pregnant there, BUDDY. Looks like you've been eating a little extra portion or two." He usually would say this while he was patting my stomach. I'm thinking to myself, thanks for the reminder.

I don't know why he thought this was funny. Or why it was his responsibility to point it out to the world. I don't think he blurted this out to be mean or to intentionally make me feel bad. I already knew I was fat; I didn't need anyone stating the obvious.

Like I mentioned, our family gatherings are typically a lot of fun. However, after putting on an extra hundred pounds, every time I get ready to go to one of these activities, I find myself thinking I would enjoy the family socials more if I weighed less.

Being fat makes social gatherings much more uncomfortable. As a fatty I found myself becoming more self conscious in any social setting. Wouldn't it be nice to go to these activities or whatever social activity I was going to and just be somewhat normal in my weight? I'm not talking about being thin, buff, six pack, eight pack or whatever, I'm just talking about being closer to a normal weight. Wouldn't I have more fun and be less self conscious?

Without a doubt, if your weight is under control, you'll feel much better at family and other social gatherings.

Wake up call!!!

In order to get and keep the right mindset, you have to be totally honest with yourself and recognize you have a problem. It took me a while to get there.

My oldest brother Rick has been a junior high mathematics teacher for over twenty years. Teaching that age group is extremely challenging. Teaching and having five teenagers in the house at one point in time, really stressed Rick out. So, he ate a lot of food for comfort. Specifically, ice cream, candy, and anything else he could get his hands on. He became about 160 pounds overweight.

So I can look at my brother, and it's easy for me to say, gee what a fatty. Trust me, the man is fat; definitely qualified as a big boy. I look at him and think, why the heck doesn't my fat brother quit eating; geez.

So, I'm at a family party and another brother, who was also overweight at the time, makes some comment about how fat Rick and I are, and he pats our stomachs, like wow you guys are really fat. So my immediate thought is; how can he make a comparison between my big fat brother and me? Hah!

So later that night I ask my wife about it and in a kind and loving way she spills the beans. "Why, yes honey, you are as fat as he is and in fact you might even be a bit larger than he is."

What, how is this possible? My brother is really fat. Could I really be that fat and maybe a little fatter? That really hurt. So, why did I lie to myself about being fat? I look in the mirror every day. I still don't understand why I had such a hard time processing the fact I had a serious weight issue.

It's like the story about cooking a live frog. You can put a frog in a pan of cold water on a stove and slowly turn up the heat and the frog will stay put until it's cooked. If you put the same frog into boiling water, he'll jump right out.

When I first started putting on weight, no one noticed, not even me. Week by week, pound by pound, the changes weren't that noticeable. Then one day, 130 pounds later, people start to notice. I'm as fat as my huge brother. I've been cooked!!!

Writing my own story became a good way to be totally honest with myself. As I read and re-

read my stories, I became even more determined to find a way to change my eating and exercise habits and achieve my ideal weight. Finally acknowledging that I had a serious weight problem was a good first step for me in developing the right mindset for a permanent lifestyle change. But it took time for me to take the next important steps.

I don't know why we think other people are heavy and overlook the fact that we are too. Now comes the dilemma; my wife has clearly been honest with me, in a loving way, but she has let me know that I am in fact as chunky as my brother. Some of you might remember the famous song, "He Ain't Heavy; He's My Brother." In this case, he is heavy, he is my brother, and he is four inches taller than I am. On a percentage basis, I am probably bigger than he is. Wow! So what have I done with this newly discovered bit of information? You're probably thinking that finally Bob has acknowledged the fact that he is a fat boy and is doing something about it. That would seem like the most logical thing to do. Unfortunately, we are not quite yet to the part in the story where "They Lived Happily Ever After." Not yet. In fact, things got worse for me, not better.

What did I do with this new found information about me being overweight? Surely knowing that I need to lose a few pounds will motivate me to get going. Sometimes it takes more than recognition. Nevertheless, being honest about your weight problem and willing to acknowledge that fact are good steps toward a solid weight loss mindset. I hope you'll relate to some of the mistakes I've made even after recognizing that I was overweight.

After realizing again, that I needed to lose some weight, I started to *get ready* to lose weight. Getting ready to lose weight has not been a good thing. How many of you have started your diet on Monday? How many Mondays have you said, "Today is the day." How many times have you said, "No more bad food. No more lying around the house. Today I will start my exercise program and I will stick to it like no other." I am sure that the medical profession has a cool sounding term for this type of behavior, to which I say, "Whatever."

The point is most of us continue to start over and over and over again. I was probably doing better without thinking about losing weight than I have by 'starting on Monday.' Whatever day of the week you decide to start losing weight, that is the best day to start. Over my 35 years of being an adult, I have probably lost hundreds of pounds; starting, stopping, and putting on more each time. Getting ready to start losing weight has not been very kind to me.

See if you relate to this process: I am going to eat everything I want this week, or this day, because soon I will begin my weight loss program, so I had better enjoy the moment. Let's see. Does this sound like the idea of eat, drink and be merry? The sad truth of the matter is that I am literally taking years off my life one bite at a time. They say that you can in fact, eat an elephant one bite at a time. However, just because you can eat the elephant, doesn't mean that you have to eat all of the elephant including the parts that are not healthy for you.

For years, whenever we ate out, I would not have a dessert with a meal. Not because I didn't like desserts, but because I was full. However, when I began 'getting ready' to lose weight, I began eating desserts even after a huge dinner. Why? Because I'd better enjoy it now before I start eating right or I will never eat a dessert again.

One of my favorite things to do while I was getting ready to lose weight was baking cookies. I've baked a mean chocolate chip cookie ever since I was in the 5th grade. Believe me, there is nothing wrong with baking cookies. It's the number that you bake and eat; that's the problem. I usually bake a double batch, so that my wife and family get to have some cookie dough and a few cookies before Dad takes over and eats 80% of the cookies. My family is cool about my chocolate chip cookie habit since I make a double batch. They don't harass me or kid around with me at all. I eat at least 10-15 cookies the night that I bake them. Is this a problem?

What am I thinking? That is a lot of cookies, especially if you have been eating some of the dough as well, which I do. OK; I know this sounds like a confession about some of my bad eating habits, it is!!

At times it seemed like I was always getting ready to lose weight. At the rate that I was 'getting ready' I might drop over and die at any moment. While I was getting ready, I would eat anything and everything I wanted fearing that I might never eat these delicious, fatty foods again. That was probably true; looking at the types of foods I used to eat.

Once while I was getting ready to start eating right, I got sick. Can't start on days like that. Then a birthday party comes up; cake and ice cream; can't miss out on that. I'll start after the birthday. I live in Utah, so you can't start eating better and exercising in July because of all the holidays. I probably have a good reason for not starting to eat and exercise right for just about every month of the year.

This 'get ready' to lose weight attitude definitely indicates that your mindset is not in place. I have done this many times over the years when I decided to lose some weight. Not any more. Finally, after developing the right mindset, I can lose weight when I want, how fast I want, and do it in a healthy smart way without starving myself. No more, "I'll start tomorrow." I'll start today if I need to and stay 'on it.' You can develop the same mindset by following the steps in this book. The principles work.

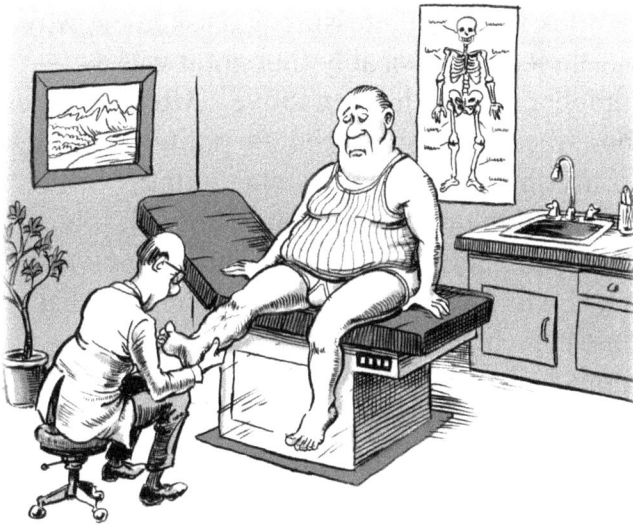

Going to the Doctor

I had a couple of dark colored moles on my
back that concerned my wife so she had me
schedule an appointment with our doctor. I like
my doctor; he is a good man who has the best
bedside manner I have ever known in the
medical profession. He takes the time to talk
with me about what's going on and offers
kindly advice.

After arriving at the office and checking in, the
assistant had me stand on the scale. Three
hundred pounds on a person who is 5'9" is not a

pretty sight. She led me back to a room, where she took my blood pressure and asked me why I was there. She probably thought it was a miracle that I could even move. After I told her about the moles, she asked me politely to take off my shirt and sit on the edge of the examination table. She then left, thankfully, closing the door behind her. The doctor walked in as I was pulling off my shirt. I'm sure that must have been one of the most frightening things he had seen all day. But ever the diplomat, he just had me sit on the edge of the examination bed, looked at the moles, said they were fine and sent me off.

Another experience with a doctor began in July when we went to a rodeo in a small town called Oakley. I grew up in a farming community. We rode horses, gathered eggs, weeded gardens, milked cows, etc. But I never got into bull riding--didn't look like much fun to me. That being said, bull riding is fun to watch. So off we went to the rodeo. As I got out of the car, the calf of my leg began hurting like no other. This pain had been coming and going for some time now, but I believed it would get better. You have to do quite a bit of walking to find your seats at the rodeo. I'm tough. I'll make it. But I'll tell ya, walking was a problem because it hurt like the dickens. Really, I could barely walk on my leg, so I had to hobble around like an injured, overweight cowboy. Not that anyone would mistake me for a cowboy. Most cowboys I know are lean and mean. I was anything but lean since I was about 140 pounds overweight. I was also wearing gym shoes and a baseball hat. Not your standard cowboy look. I went home barely able to walk.

Over the course of the next three and a half weeks, the pain in my leg refused to get better. I tried to rub it out, walk it out; I tried everything I could think of to find some relief from the pain. I should have gone to the doctor.

One night the pain became so intense my hands were trembling. I decided it was time to see a doctor. My doctor was out of town so I saw the doctor on call. He told me just what I wanted to hear and what many doctors say when you first go in with a problem. "It's probably nothing; I'll prescribe a painkiller for you and if it continues to hurt come back."

Wow! Thanks for the help (really?). I'm not buying it this time! "Let's be on the safe side and get the leg scanned."

To his credit, he ordered the scan and it was done within a couple of hours. I'm sure he thought the scan would be clean and the pain medication would be sufficient. Unfortunately, the scan showed a DVT, a very serious type of blood clot that had developed in the back of my knee.

Preventing further damage to my leg required some drastic and expensive measures. First of all I had two shots a day in the stomach with something called Lovenox. I don't know much about it but it stings like crazy and it's expensive. For the ten shots I had, it was about $1400. Believe me, this was not a lot of fun. Here it was the middle of summer, we had a boating trip planned and the family reunion was coming up. This was not the time to have a blood clot.

The doctor told me to keep the leg elevated for two to four weeks so the veins could reform around the clot. At the end of four weeks my leg continued to feel better if it was elevated. Sitting down and walking caused excruciating pain. Here's the fun thing about having a blood clot, you look completely healthy, and therefore, you get no sympathy.

I can't help but wonder if I could have avoided this whole nightmare if I had eaten the right kind of foods and stayed in shape. A blood clot can happen to anyone anytime, but wouldn't my chances be better for avoiding these kinds of health issues if I were eating right and staying active? We may never know, but why test fate?

Even after dealing with this clot, I still didn't have the right mindset for losing weight.

If I could turn back the clock and avoid this health problem I would. But what about today, what about tomorrow? What health issues can I avert if I get into shape and begin eating right?

This has truly been one of the most trying health problems I have ever had. Isn't it time to make the necessary changes in my lifestyle so that I won't be forced to do it later? If you don't have your health, life is tough and not as fulfilling. What has a higher priority than getting and staying healthy?

It's not too late for me to change my eating and exercise habits and improve the quality of my life. I'm still here; my leg is healing; I still have a lot of things I want to do in life. If I learn from this experience and share it with others, it also reminds me of how important it is to eat right and stay in shape. Learn from the past, focus on today and plan for a better tomorrow.

Is Exercise Enough???

After I had my little run in with the blood clot, I decided to find a gym and start exercising regularly. I have been doing some light weight lifting along with some walking. It has helped how I feel and made a big difference in my ability to do basic things, such as bend over, put on shoes etc.

I used to think that exercise was all you had to do to lose weight. But, don't kid yourself. For most of us professional eaters who are overweight, just working out is not going to be enough. That's right folks. Work your guts out at the gym, but if you don't reel in the eating habits, you will not get the results that you want.

Realize that if you are ever going to permanently overcome your weight problem, *changing your eating habits is absolutely essential.*

Changing habits is not easy to do but with the right mindset, anything is possible and life can be amazing along the way. You are going to feel so awesome once you start down the path and begin to see results.

Monday, a New Beginning?

How many times have you decided to start your weight loss plan on Monday?

This is yet another huge obstacle for weight loss success. You know this one, and like me, you have been guilty of this one over and over again. How do I know? Because I have lived it and made the same mistake and I know that I am not alone on this one.

I thought I would begin exercising first, and then start eating better after my body adjusted to the weightlifting and walking. Knowing that I was going to start eating healthy foods soon (soon being the relative term), I decided I should eat anything and everything I wanted.

I should eat all my favorite foods before beginning my new eating program (by the truckloads). Now I know I am not alone in this particular concept. Most of us, (who are honest with ourselves), have done this. Hey, I'm going to start eating better on Monday, so this weekend I had better eat like crazy; roast beef, mashed potatoes, ice-cream, popcorn, etc. Eat, drink and be merry for on Monday I begin to eat better! Ha!! Isn't that a laugh? We all know what a farce that idea is because when Monday rolls around, we easily justify why Monday won't work. Perhaps I need to go shopping first. This week I have several appointments that involve eating out. So, really there's not much point to working at it this week, so I'll start a week from Monday. That gives me plenty of time for more good food and getting ready.

Isn't it nice to have Monday as the designated start day? That way if we blow it on Monday, or Tuesday, (usually it's all over for me by noon on Monday), we just skip it for the rest of the week. I can make another run at it next Monday.

Do you know how many Monday's I have committed to start eating better? I'm not sure that I can even count that high. I can tell you for a certainty, that I have been ready to rock and roll next Monday so many times it is almost unbelievable. Occasionally, I have made it through the lunch hour, but when I get home that night, there it is, left over roast beef, mashed potatoes, and gravy served on bread, yum. Then to make sure that I got enough fat grams, let's have two or three chocolate sundaes. Ohhhh, I am so glad that I am not starting on Monday now and I am so glad that I can put off starting again until next Monday. Now, I can continue to eat all my favorite foods all week long. One more weekend to really go at it because I am going to start eating better on what day? Yep, on Monday, a whole week away.

So the problem in a nutshell is that exercise is only part of what you need to do to lose weight. Controlling your eating habits is perhaps even more important.

Today is the day to eat right and exercise. I would suggest you start any day but Monday. You're sure to have more success. Try starting on Thursday; it worked much better for me.

.

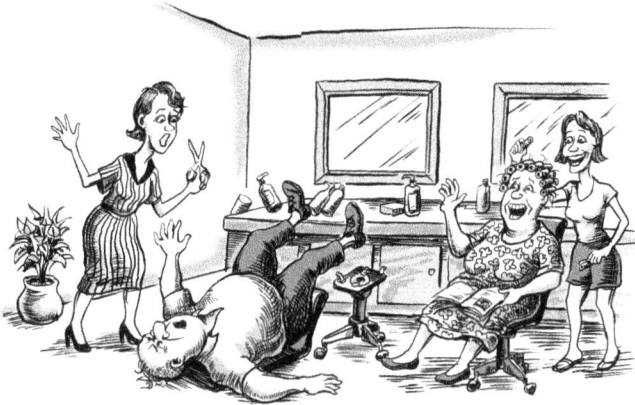

Going to the Barber

Getting a haircut was always a 'big' concern for me. Squeezing into the chair and sitting my enormous bulk down between the arm rests, I felt like the chair would break in two and dump me out on the floor at any moment. Will getting up be possible? Will I survive the tumble?

If I live, I'm sure that it's going to be an interesting event. Janette, who cuts my hair, is very kind and doesn't say anything, but I'm sure she's checked her insurance policy to be sure she's covered for such an event. Won't that make great gossip for the neighborhood. 'Big Bob takes fall, busts salon chair in half.'

Do you think I should have to be worrying about such a thing? Truly, a proud moment.

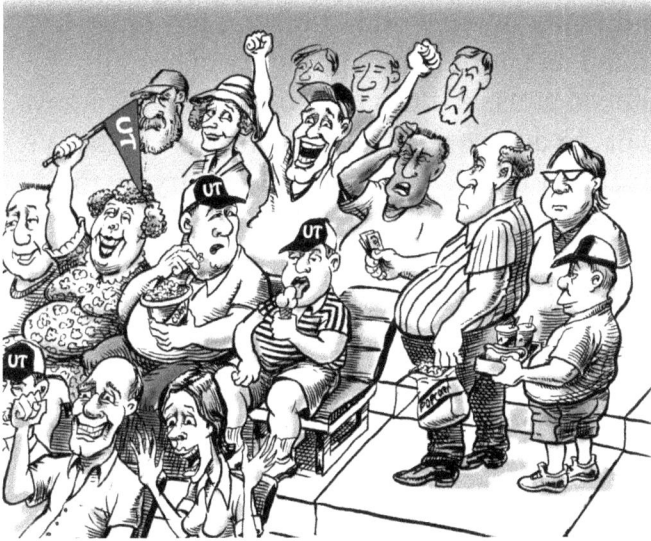

Finding a Place to Sit

My family occasionally enjoys attending
football games. Naturally, I get our seats next
to the aisle, avoiding seats in the center of the
row which are a hard to get to for fat people.
Good thinking Bob, now we won't have to
climb over everybody. We park the car, make
the long hike to the stadium, climb the stairs
and begin looking for our seats. We find the
row where our seats are located, but three of our
four seats are already taken. There is only one
of our four seats available. I look down the row

assessing the problem and realize I am not the
only fatty in the world. In fact, I have just
found an entire family of fatties. They all
looked at us as if to say, "sorry, we don't know
what to do, we need the room." Here was a
bunch of fatties, including myself, trying to fit
into stadium seats not designed for fatties.
Believe me, they were fat. Being a fellow fatty,
I didn't really want to say too much, and frankly
I felt bad for them. There were eleven fat men
and women taking up fourteen seats including
three of our four seats. They all scrunched
together trying desperately to free up our three
seats but to no avail. No matter how much they
scrunched, they were only able to free up two of
our four seats. There were four of us, and of
course, we paid big bucks for these tickets. So,
to solve the problem, two of them had to sit in
the aisle to free up our spots.

Tragically, here I am, a big time fatty myself,
waiting for them to free up our spots. I really
felt bad for them and for myself. My children,
who were younger and smaller, didn't take up
as much seat space. That left plenty of room for
me to sit. Otherwise, I would have been sitting
in the aisle with my other two fat friends or
doing the half-on-the-seat straddle.

When going to restaurants, movies or other
events, do you have a hard time finding seating?

As a fat person finding a seat is sometimes very difficult for me.

Whenever we go to a restaurant as a family, the tactful waitress asks if a booth is ok. Most of the time we can find a booth with a table that has a side that fits fat people or is movable. You might call them fat compatible booths with movable tables. Not all eating booths are created equal. I learned this after years of personal and sad experience. Mercifully, most booths at a restaurant either have a movable table that I can shift, creating enough room for my bulk, or there is enough room for me to squeeze in and fit relatively well on one side or the other. Many times, depending on the restaurant, I will flat out request a table where I can shift the chair so I can sit comfortably.

Imagine this though. You are in a restaurant that has fairly tight booths. All of the tables are full and the only place available to sit is in a booth. What do you say? "Uh, can we wait for a fat compatible booth please?"

When I go out to eat with a business associate or a friend, I have to quickly eyeball the size of the booth, determine if the table is movable or has a side big enough for the fat guy. If my friend or acquaintance sits down first, taking the 'fat side' then I tactfully find a way to change seats. "Uh, excuse me; I need the side with a little more room, please." Awkward!

Wouldn't eating out at a restaurant be more pleasant if I didn't have to worry about the size of the booth?

Rick, my older brother and I are both restaurant booth challenged. We like to go to the buffet for 'business meetings.' We have collaborated from time to time on work related projects. During some summers while he is not teaching, he works a little for my company part time in the real estate business. One summer we would meet almost every Monday for lunch to talk about business and starting a diet, 'next Monday.' One of our favorite places (which should come as no surprise to fat folks) was the all-you-can-eat buffet. Is there a better place to hold a three hour meeting than at an 'all-you-can-eat buffet?' We would talk a little business but certainly our main focus was the food. After eating a huge meal and going back for seconds and sometime thirds, I could still eat eight or ten cookies, plus ice cream and cake for dessert. You simply would not believe how much I could eat.

Rick was no slacker either. He easily kept up with me. He would eat a huge salad with mushrooms, hard-boiled eggs, raisins, and lettuce with ranch dressing. Then he'd go back for chicken, potatoes, rice, beans, and squash. Then he'd go back again. Then before leaving, he'd get plenty of cake, brownies, and ice cream. I don't know if he ate more than me but I'd like to think so.

I'm sure that when the owners and cooks saw us coming, they wondered if they could keep up with the demand. They may have hired an extra accountant to make sure we weren't affecting the buffets' bottom line too much, no pun intended. To be sure, we always got our money's worth.

Looking back, I get a kick out of our seating arrangements at the buffet. Rick did not like to do the dining tables in the main area of the buffet, which always work better for those of us who are 'booth challenged.' The seats at the tables have hard backs so he preferred the cushions that you could lean against in the booths. We couldn't sit at just any booth; we had to sit in a corner booth where there was a movable table that would accommodate our enormous sizes. We couldn't really sit across from each other because we were too fat, so we sat kitty-corner to one another, the only way we could comfortably sit in a booth.

But really, how pathetic is that, to only have a couple of corner booths in the whole restaurant where we could sit.

I can remember going to the buffet with him on a particularly busy day and checking out the corner booths in several rooms and finding them taken. We had to settle for a table. Sitting at a table was not fun for my brother. Seriously, I can't believe that we put ourselves in this position. When you stop and think about it, being fat prevents you from living a normal life. Wouldn't it be nice if Rick and I could sit comfortably at any booth?

How about fat people at the movies? I make sure I get there in plenty of time so I can get an aisle seat. Because if I don't, I'll be sitting somewhere in the middle and you know what that means. Some of the newer theatres in the valley have systems where you can purchase tickets and reserve your seats in advance. What a great innovation for those of us who need an aisle.

My family likes sitting in the center seats of the theatre for a better view of the screen. I like to buy pop and popcorn at the movies. However, when I do, guess what happens in the middle of the show? "Excuse me sir, sorry ma'am."

And what are the other movie patrons saying and thinking; "Hey, watch the feet!" "Get your fat behind out of my face!" "We're trying to see a movie here!"

I really hate crawling over people to get in and out. It's embarrassing. Such a simple little thing like finding a seat in a movie theatre can become a big deal when you're overweight.

Going to social and public events would be more relaxing and fun if we were at a more comfortable weight, don't you think?

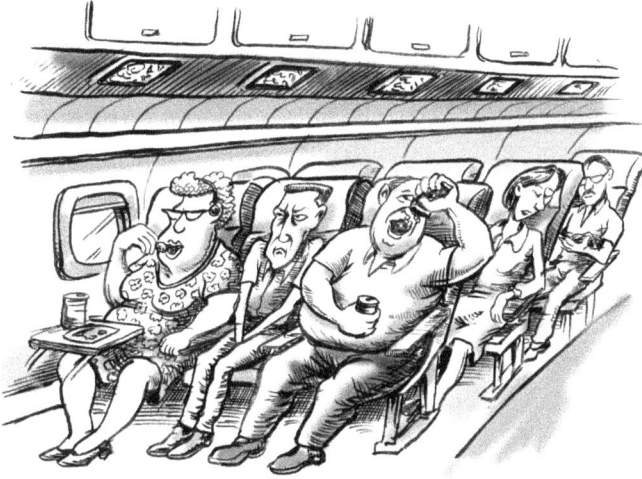

The Airplane Ride

My brother Rick has taught junior high for
many years. He sometimes blames his eating
habits on this stressful profession but really it's
no excuse and he knows it. He's in the process
of writing his own story and he let me share this
one with you.

Rick boarded a 747 on his way back from a
short trip out of town. On the way to his seat,
he noticed that the other gentleman in his row,
like himself, was also a rather stout man.
Lucky for them they were assigned seats A and

C and no one was assigned to sit in between them. Now really, who was the lucky one? Believe me, the lucky one was the guy that didn't have to sit between these two men. Someone out there has no idea just how lucky he was that this flight was not particularly crowded. Sitting in between these two beauties would not have been fun.

Rick sat down in his seat and introduced himself. As the engine revved up, the stewardess began the preflight litany with the standard presentation, "In case of loss in cabin pressure, be sure to put on your air mask first, then help others around you, use your seat as a flotation device if you crash in water, (good luck with that one), don't barf on the floor, use the bag etc. And lastly, here's how your seat belt works," (my personal favorite).

Before takeoff fastening the seat belt is required. My brother and his stout friend attempted to put on their seat belts--normally, not a big deal. However, neither of them could buckle their seat belts. Here are these very big men doing everything they can to fasten their safety belts. Finally, they gave up and looked at each other. My brother said, "Now what?" relieved he wasn't the only one having the belt issue.

Now what? Raise your hand and announce to the whole plane full of people that your seat belt won't buckle. Let the whole world know right now, once and for all, that these ridiculous seat belts were made too small. Yep, the manufacturer obviously made a mistake. He hadn't accounted for the fact that two baby whales would somehow board this plane and need a seat belt larger than normal. Shame on that engineer, what was he thinking?

Rick and his seating companion shrugged their shoulders and did nothing--nothing wrong with that choice. However, I have heard of flights where the plane suddenly dropped and if you didn't have your seat belt on, your head hit the ceiling. People have actually gone flying in the air. I have personally been on some pretty rough flights but none where the people went sailing through the air. When my brother told me this story, one of my first thoughts was, what if something had gone wrong with the flight? Then I thought, well Rick and his traveling friend would probably have been fine regardless of what happened. These two were so tightly wedged into their seats no amount of turbulence or storm would have forced them out of their seats. Who needs a seat belt when you can wedge yourself in between the arm rests? They were lucky to wedge themselves into a single seat.

I've heard of some airlines considering treating overweight people like extra luggage and charging by the pound. This could be quite costly for some folks.

Flying would certainly be easier and more enjoyable for all involved if we took up just a little less space, wouldn't you agree?

Start Writing Your Own Story

Writing my own story became a good way to be totally honest with myself. As I read and re-read my stories, I became more determined to find a way to change my eating and exercise habits and achieve my ideal weight.

I suggest you go to your workbook and begin writing examples from your life that illustrate what you want to change. Or you can begin your list of 'whys.'

Perhaps the most important factor in determining how strong your mindset becomes is how well you write your own story and how powerful your 'whys' are. Be patient, take time with it, and learn how to ask yourself the right questions. Why do you want to change your eating and exercise habits? How will your life improve? What will be better about your new lifestyle? Why do you want to lose weight? Add to your stories and your list of 'whys' throughout the **5-Minute Mindset** process.

Writing my own story made all the difference for me. It provided me with powerful personal reasons for improving and staying with my plan. Any time I began to falter I could go back to my story and remind myself why weight loss was important to me. Writing my own story gave me the necessary momentum needed for developing the right mindset for long-term weight loss success.

I spent much of my time in this area in preparation for my weight loss program. As I mentioned before, losing 73 pounds in five months took a powerful mindset and writing my own story was a major factor of that success.

I also found that using creativity in writing my story such as designing the cartoons helped me express my weight loss concerns in a unique way and was something I enjoyed doing.

Additionally, I found that sharing my stories and 'whys' with others helped me develop the right mindset.

Begin writing your story today.

Step 3
Set Your Goals

Setting your weight loss goals is the next step. Setting specific, achievable goals is essentially the first step in designing a plan, which we cover more fully in Step 4. However, setting your weight loss goals is critical to your plan and so important to your success, that it is included here as a separate step. You will be better prepared for this step by completing steps one and two of the **5-Minute Mindsetting** process. Make sure you have some powerful 'whys' in place as you begin setting your goals.

Deciding that weight loss is a priority and establishing powerful 'why's' form the foundation of the mindsetting process. As you practice and implement the nine **5-Minute Mindsetting** steps, you will change your eating and exercise habits for the better.

When you set your goals, write them down and plan on reviewing them daily. Make sure that your goals are specific and achievable. Break your goals down to yearly, monthly, weekly and daily goals. As you set your goals make sure they reflect what you really want. Make the decision to never give in to setbacks, discouragement or a change in circumstance. Never quit, and never give up! "Keep trying until the difficult becomes possible, the possible becomes a habit and the habits become who you are" (Dieter Uchtdorf 2009).

How quickly do you want to complete the **5-Minute Mindsetting** process and begin losing weight? What specifically do you want to achieve? Go into detail on this step and write it down in your workbook. The workbook provides you with a step by step process for setting goals. Have both short and long term goals. Where do you want to be five years from now; one year from now; a month from now; a week from now; tomorrow?

Your goals should be achievable. When I first set my weight loss goal, I set it for what I weighed when I was 21. I felt this would be a nice weight for me. After more thought, I decided to lower that expectation.

Make your goals incremental and suited to your capacities. Even though I weigh myself every day, I don't worry about the daily fluctuations. I pay attention to the overall weekly progress.

It is best if you write your goals down.
However, if you mentally keep track of your
goals and review them daily, this will still yield
positive results. Also, realize that as you take
action on your goals, other ideas and solutions
to your unique challenges will surface. Make
adjustments as needed.

You don't necessarily have to wait until your
goals are completely written down in every
detail before you begin to take action. For
example, you may decide to lose thirty pounds
and that drinking skim milk instead of 2%
might help; go ahead and begin. Don't wait for
a full plan. Take action now!

I recommend that you think about and review
your goals daily. Make a decision to stay the
course no matter what. Measure and account
for the goal every day. Stay focused on your
goals. Why are they important to you? How
will it feel as you achieve them and make the
wanted changes in your life? Keep the goals
simple. For example, your goal might be 'by
the end of the next six months, I want to weigh
150 pounds.' Notice that the goal includes a
deadline and a specific weight target. From this
goal you can set some monthly intermediate
goals. As you achieve your daily and monthly
goals your self esteem and self respect will
grow.

Challenges that get you off track will come.
The key is to review your goals and account for
them daily in your workbook or journal.
Reviewing your goals daily takes just minutes.
Do it and get results. Remember and see the
big picture and realize that daily battles, won or
lost, may or may not win the war.

As you take action on your goals, your mindset
will get stronger and carry you through difficult
moments when you are tempted to veer off your
chosen path. All of us have set goals and failed
again and again. For some, setting goals has
become a trite phrase with little meaning.

The **5-Minute Mindsetting** process is unique
and dynamic, strengthening your resolve and
commitment to the weight loss process.

With the **5-Minute Mindset**, you make an
absolute commitment to do whatever it takes to
reach the destination in mind. With the right
mindset about your goals, there can be no
failure, only success. You might lose a battle
here and there but you choose not to give up,
you choose to keep going and win the war.
Every day you are closer to the dream and the
vision you want to achieve.

As you make an absolute commitment to lose weight, the necessary resources begin to surface. You've decided your weight loss goal is something you want to achieve and you are willing to pay whatever price must be paid to achieve it. You will find others interested in similar goals and who are willing to help.

Throughout history there are examples of men and women who set goals and achieved them through a powerful mindset. One of these was Cortez. Cortez, upon landing in the new world was confronted by a nation of hundreds of thousands of natives; many were fierce and cunning warriors.

When confronted by the challenge to conquer the land, some of his men wanted to return home to Spain. Cortez made the decision to stay and conquer the land for Spain. He burned his own ships that lay in the bay waiting to take them home to safety.

With a few cannons, some horses, and circumstances that played into the Spaniards' hands, they conquered the Aztecs and won glory for the Spanish Crown. The course of history in the Americas was changed forever.

American history is filled with examples of men and women who developed a powerful mindset.

You might read some of their stories as an aid in developing yours.

You know stories of other men and women whose visions and dreams came to fruition because of determination, work, and faith. There is no reason why you can't write a story of your own; a story of determination, courage, and hope.

After establishing powerful 'whys' setting goals is perhaps the second most important step in the **5-Minute Mindsetting** process.   Men like Columbus, Cortez, George Washington and Abraham Lincoln had powerful 'whys' in place as they worked to achieve goals for themselves and their countries.

The challenges we face in our own personal lives may not be as dramatic or as great as the men mentioned. But, the future of our lives and the lives of those we love may very well be impacted by the choices we make today and how we choose to face our difficulties and challenges. Developing a powerful mindset may make the difference between our success or failure in achieving our goals.

Every day I fed my mind with ideas and thoughts about my goals. By doing so, I was able to strengthen my mindset and generate daily, weekly and monthly strategies which enabled me to form new habits and change the way I ate and exercised.

After choosing to lose weight, I decided to lose 120 pounds over the course of 12 months. I broke that down to 10 pounds per month. I spent a few minutes every day thinking about this goal and what I would do that day toward achieving that goal. Every day I had a plan and followed it.

Make sure to check with a physician as to what your target weight should be and how fast you can safely lose weight. You can find a lot of information and additional resources online as you think about your weight loss goals.

Workbook Assignment: Write down how much weight you want to lose. Break this goal down into weekly and monthly goals. Set deadlines. Make a commitment to review these goals daily.

Step 4
Design a Plan

After setting your weight loss goals, you are ready to design a plan for achieving them. Your plan consists of a set of weight loss habits that you are going to implement in achieving your goals. Your goals and plans form a map that will guide you to your desired results. Your plan or map is an important part for achieving your weight loss goals.

How important is your plan? It is essential! No one would start a fifty-mile hike without a solid plan. The type of terrain you'll be traversing determines the type of footwear you'll wear. How much food and water will you need to take or where along the path will you have an opportunity to stop for food and water?

Would you start a vacation without thinking about the type of transportation you were going to use and how much time it will take to make the trip? What tourist attractions do you want to see? How much will it cost for the trip?

Do you think spending time planning is important? How long have you been overweight? How long have you been overeating and less active than you should be? Spending quality time designing a plan and preparing for your program will pay big dividends.

As you decide on a habit that needs to change, think about how to do it. Make a list of these ideas; this becomes your plan. Begin implementing these ideas immediately. For example, I decided to cut down on my fat gram intake. I did this by paying attention to the fat content of the foods I ate. I immediately implemented this plan and saw results.

As you design your plan there are three fundamental principles to keep in mind: **develop a powerful mindset, eat healthier, and be more active.**

I developed my plan keeping these fundamental principles in mind. All of the ideas presented in this step fit in one or more of the above categories. As you implement your plan, if you do not get the results you want, then make adjustments in one or more of these areas.

My plan consists of a few basic rules that I review and do every day. They are based on years of observation and trial and error. These ideas should help you as you design your customized weight loss program.

As you develop your weight loss strategies, implement them as you go. The sooner you begin getting results and achieving your goals, the stronger your mindset will become. Let your plan evolve as you take action.

Develop a Powerful Mindset

I began my most recent weight loss effort by developing a powerful mindset first. Going through this process was the single most important thing that I did and has been the difference between long and short term success. Your mindset develops as you implement the principles discussed in this book. Your plan should consist of reviewing your story, your goals, and the actions you must take to achieve your goals. Creating a workable plan is a process and takes time, how long, is up to you.

My brother's wife, using this system, began working on her mindset. She made a plan, implemented it and within two weeks, lost ten pounds. My brother at the time of this writing has lost fifty pounds over a period of five months.

By reading this book, thinking about all the principles contained in it and becoming actively involved in your own weight loss program, you will begin developing the mindset needed to accomplish your weight loss goals. If you have done the steps as outlined so far, you are already on the path to having the right mindset.

Eat Healthier

I developed a simple eating plan that worked for my lifestyle. Everyone's plan will be a little different and that's OK. Whatever your plan is, once you implement it, stay with it--keep working at it--let it evolve.

My plan consists of the following guidelines.

General Guidelines for Breakfast, Lunch, Dinners and Snacks

1. Drink water, juice or lemonade instead of carbonated drinks. Use low fat milk.
2. Don't eat fries, onion rings or any other deep fried foods.
3. Eat more fruits and vegetables.
4. Eat more chicken and fish either grilled or baked. Avoid deep fried or breaded meats.

5. Eat less beef and pork. If you have beef or pork, make sure it is grilled or baked.
6. When snacking, eat low fat or no fat cookies, candy, popcorn, etc.
7. Use low fat butter in place of margarine or real butter.
8. Buy only low fat frozen dinners. Fat gram content will vary widely from brand to brand.
9. Eat pancakes, and cereals with lower fat content.
10. Eat bacon and breads with lower fat content.
11. Don't starve yourself. Eat or snack as necessary within the guidelines. Have fruits and vegetables or other healthy snacks on hand – avoid hunger pains.
12. Replace high fat ice-cream with low fat ice cream or frozen yogurt.
13. Eat until you're satisfied, not stuffed. Don't finish everything on your plate just because it's there.
14. Be sure to drink lots of water.

Guidelines for Eating Out

I have a very busy lifestyle and eat out a lot-- this has been one of my biggest weight loss challenges. But here's something I learned; you can eat out, enjoy it, and still lose weight. Here is the key.

I know ahead of time exactly what I can order and stay within my plan. My plan helps me decide before hand what I can eat. My mindset helps me stick to the plan, even when I am tempted to go back to my old habits. Passing up unhealthy foods is easy for me today because of a solid plan and mindset.

1. Eat more chicken and fish either grilled or baked. Avoid deep fried or breaded meats.
2. Eat less beef and pork. If you have beef or pork make sure it is grilled or baked.
3. Plan in advance where you are going to eat, what you are going to eat and stick to it.
4. Check out the fat gram content in fast food meals before eating there (online).
5. Be flexible when eating out with others but watch your portions. Stay within the general guidelines as much as possible.
6. Share with your friends and family your new eating habits. This will help them when deciding where to eat.
7. Avoid mayonnaise, fry sauce, and other high in fat condiments. Check the fat content on all sauces by checking for this information online (you'll be surprised).
8. When tempted to order a carbonated drink, order a non-carbonated drink instead. There are other choices; fruit punch, lemonade, juices, etc.

9. Plan on taking part of the meal home as leftovers for another meal.
10. Check fat content in breads and rolls. Avoid restaurant butter.
11. Use low fat dressings or vinaigrette on salads.
12. At 'all you can eat' restaurants, spend plenty of time at the salad and fruit bar.

Be More Active--My Exercise Plan

I walk forty to fifty minutes a day six days a week. I lift weights about 40 minutes three days a week on Mondays, Wednesdays, and Fridays.

Becoming more active can include activities like swimming, running, walking or other aerobic activities. The idea is to get more active and burn calories. In general, work up to staying consistently active for 40 minutes or longer.

It's important as you develop your weight loss plan that you include both an exercise and an eating component. Changing both your eating and exercise habits will maximize the results of your plan.

When I decided to start losing weight, I already had an exercise plan in place. Before I began

losing weight consistently, I had to change my
eating habits as well.

I am a big fan of exercising. When I began my
weight loss program, I began with the exercise
component. I went to the gym and worked out
five days a week. I lifted weights and walked.
As I continued to exercise, I felt better and
stronger, but I didn't begin losing weight until I
changed my eating habits, then the results were
dramatic. I learned that an effective exercise
and eating program can result in significant,
rapid weight loss. How much and how rapid
the loss depends on your goals, mindset, and
plan.

Keep Your Plan Simple and Achievable

Your plan may be as simple as my niece's plan.
She learned that in order to lose two pounds a
week she had to keep her calorie intake between
1400 to 1800 calories per day. She found this
information online. She began counting
calories and lost 30 pounds in three months.

In her plan, she allows herself what she calls
one cheat day per week. She found that this had
a number of benefits for her. It gave her a
better attitude toward eating right. She's an
active mother with three children. Finding time
to exercise is very challenging. She found that

sticking to eating good foods and reducing portions is enough for achieving her goals. She has found an exercise program that fits into her busy schedule and has added that to her plan.

My brother's wife loves sweets. She is unwilling to totally give them up, but as part of her plan, she allows herself a small low calorie treat each night if she has stayed within her plan during the day. She continues to be very successful losing the weight she wants.

My brother is also a great lover of sweets, but now instead of thinking about a candy bar when he gets a sweet tooth, he thinks about how good a few grapes or some watermelon would be.

After reading my weight loss guidelines, eliminating carbonated drinks became an important part of my brother's plan, but he really likes carbonated drinks. In order to solve this dilemma, he began looking for tasty drink replacements like light lemonades to take the place of his carbonated drinks. This has worked out very well in his plan.

Part of my plan also included ways to deal with my love of candy, ice cream and sugar. I found sweets that were low in fat content that fit into my plan and I decided when I would allow myself to eat these sweets. It takes time to develop the right eating habits and form the right mindset for a lasting change.

My brother and I are very different in the ways we approached our weight loss plans. My brother chose to count the calories and fat in the foods he was eating. My plan is to know the fat gram content of food generally and eat those that contain less fat.

Wrapping It Up

As you design your eating and exercise plans, remember your reasons for changing your habits—it really works. Review your 'whys'. Review your plans and goals daily. Doing this just a few minutes a day strengthens your mindset and reminds you of the strategies you will employ during the day in accomplishing your goals.

Now it's important to organize and prioritize your ideas and research into your own customized weight loss plan. What hard and fast rules are you going to make for yourself that can facilitate your success? What steps do you need to take to achieve your ideal weight? Keep your plan simple and achievable. Memorize it or write it down in your workbook.

Step 5
Implement the Plan

Implementing the plan means taking action. You have already taken action towards developing your **5-Minute Mindset** by purchasing this book, making a decision, writing your own story, setting your goals, and designing your plan. You have identified habits that you want to change and replace with new habits. Simply put, you have decided to adjust your level of activity and change your eating habits so that you can lose weight. Now it's time to be 'on it!'

Being 'On It' means that you are fully involved in achieving your plan on a daily, weekly, and monthly basis. You are keeping your commitments according to your plan. Every day before you leave the house you think about and review your goals and plan. This process should take about five minutes. You make commitments and complete the plan for the day so at the end of the day you can say, "I did it; I kept my commitments." You want to do the same thing for the week. You can't be 'on it'

until you are fully engaged in completing the
work as outlined in your plan.

There are many examples in life that reflect this
idea. Many of you have probably flown before.
When an aircraft takes off, there has to be a
flight plan. There is a pilot and a co-pilot who
checks each system to make sure the plane is
ready to fly. Take off is the most dangerous
and difficult moment for the pilots. The plane
must achieve a certain speed before lift off.
Gaining the momentum and speed necessary for
taking off requires a lot of energy and fuel.
Once the plane reaches cruising altitude, less
energy is required to keep the plane aloft.

You have found the right runway; you're,
beginning to taxi. Now you have to apply
enough energy to get the plane off the ground.

The energy you put into your previous steps is
now ready to be released by steady and
consistent action until you reach your cruising
altitude. Achieving lift off and reaching your
cruising altitude is being 'on it.'

As you take off, there could be wind sheer or
other dangerous conditions that may make the
take off difficult. Through proper preparation,
you are ready for whatever you need to do to

get the plane up. This is also part of being 'on it.'

A pilot has to be aware of the course, direction and altitude of the plane. Air controllers help pilots maintain their flight plan and stay on course to their destination. Sometimes course corrections during the flight are necessary to bring the plane to its destination. Maybe, you have to change altitude or direction to get around or above a storm. Hopefully, you have enough fuel to meet the demands. Crash landings are typically not survived.

As you think about being 'on it' and implementing your own plan, review your own story, keeping the plane analogy in mind. I think you'll find it helpful.

Whatever you choose to do, be sure to consult with a doctor or other professional whenever beginning an exercise or weight loss program.

Don't wait to buy this or that before implementing either your exercise plan or your eating plan. Just begin. You will gain confidence as you implement even part of your plan and begin to have some success. The sooner you begin having some success, the more likely you are to follow through with the rest of your plan. You've designed a plan that will form new eating and exercise habits that will change your life for the better. What commitments are you going to make today to get you going toward that better and more fulfilling lifestyle?

You're already spending some time every day reviewing and thinking about your goals. Your plan for accomplishing your goals is taking shape. You have some ideas of what you want to do and you are ready to take steady and consistent action toward achieving your focused goals. As you take steady and consistent action, you're new eating and exercise habits will begin to form. At times you may be tempted to drift from your plan because of illness or other circumstances. Remember, you have decided to lose weight; stay with it.

As you lose weight, and achieve some of your goals, your mindset is reinforced. Your weekly progress will be determined by your daily activity.

As I followed my plan consistently on a daily basis, I typically had a positive weekly result. I did not worry about daily weight fluctuations. Be careful setting daily weight loss goals. Weekly weigh-ins may also fluctuate up and down; this is not a cause for immediate concern.

If you stay 'on it,' stay focused and stick with your plan; weight loss should follow.

Here is an example of how I implement my plan on a daily basis. The first thing I do is exercise. I walk for forty minutes and spend twenty to thirty minutes either stretching or weightlifting. I lift weights three days a week and walk six days a week. As I walk, I think about and review my goals, my overall daily plan and repeat from memory inspirational thoughts or poems.

Lifting weights builds muscle that burns calories more effectively and efficiently. If you don't have a lot of money, buy some 5 to 8 lb. hand weights and start with some very simple exercises.

I'm a big fan of cardiovascular exercises which would include walking, swimming, or bicycling.

Walking is one of the easiest cardiovascular exercises you can pick up. Start small and work up gradually until you can walk at least forty minutes a day. You may have to build up to that level of exercise. Check with your physician or trainer for your personal exercise needs.

You might prefer running, swimming or riding a bike. By planning in advance what your exercise will be, the decision is already made. My daily exercise program is a habit that I enjoy doing every day.

My eating plan is simple. I keep breakfast fast and easy. Generally I eat some type of a low-fat cereal and avoid cereals with high sugar content. I use 1% or low fat milk. I also enjoy toast with my meal. Whether it's white or wheat bread makes no difference as long as it is low in fat. There are many types of low fat bread today that you can use in your diet. I personally like bread made with a variety of grains and great nutritional benefits. I also use a low fat butter rather than 'real' butter or margarine. I like my toast with jam or honey.

I also enjoy a variety of fruits with breakfast including grapes, oranges, grapefruit, and bananas.

Instead of cereal, I occasionally eat pancakes or French toast. Instead of butter, I use syrup, jams, jellies or honey instead. I also avoid using butter when cooking.

I also drink a variety of fruit juices.

The keys for my breakfasts are keep it simple, keep it fast, and keep it low in fat.

Typically I eat out for lunch because of what I do professionally. If you like fast food, you can go online and get the nutritional information and find foods that will fit in your plan. I keep the fat grams between 6 and 8. I avoid condiments that are heavy in fat, like mayonnaise, tartar sauce, and many other sauces. I check the fat gram content online for all sauces before eating at fast food restaurants. I prefer chicken and hamburger grilled rather than cooked on a flat surface.

When I eat lunch at home, I usually have a turkey or chicken sandwich with some type of fruit. I avoid the fatty condiments for all sandwiches.

Sometimes instead of sandwiches, I enjoy low fat soups with Baked Lays Potato Chips or other low fat crackers.

For dinners, the basic rules of health apply. You should eat more chicken and fish rather than steak and roast beef. A good mixture of vegetables with salads is always good. You can go online and get recipes and other ideas for low fat meals that can be easily prepared at home. Once again, I think that simplicity is the key. When the family is eating something for dinner that is too high in fat, I reduce portions and enhance my dinner with some fruit and vegetables.

Common sense is the basic principle for all healthy eating. For dinners eat foods lower in fat. Use less gravy. I prefer grilled chicken and steak rather than frying meat in a pan. Baking chicken and steak is also a healthier way to prepare these meats. When I'm pressed for time, I'll eat frozen dinners. Be sure to verify the fat grams in the dinner. Not all frozen dinners are created the same. One small dinner can have between twenty and thirty fat grams in it, while other brands will have between six and eight fat grams in the meal. Watch those fat grams.

In general, the idea is to keep it simple, use common sense and eat more fruits and vegetables.

There are also a number of desserts that you can prepare that are low in fat. You can buy low-fat brownies, low-fat cake, low-fat cream, low-fat cheese; you can even buy low-fat cream cheese.

My wife actually experimented with some of the regular recipes for cookies by substituting low fat yogurt in place of the oil; some of them turned out pretty good but some of them did not turn out so well. Don't be afraid to experiment and have some fun watching those fat grams and eating healthier.

Don't eat dinner too late at night. When you sleep, your metabolism slows down. This is a particularly sensitive subject for me, because I would eat late at night all the time. It was only through developing the right mindset that I was able to quit eating late at night.

But if you are going to eat late at night, be sure to eat the right kinds of foods like fruits, low-fat cookies, or low-fat potato chips etc.

Plan nights to splurge. I still stay with my plan of not drinking pop or eating foods loaded with fat. But occasionally, I do splurge. I eat low fat or no fat foods, just more of them. I especially enjoy a variety of fruits like grapes, apples, oranges, watermelon, honeydew, and cantaloupe.

Implementing your plan and taking action brings positive results and strengthens your mindset. Keep the implementation of your plan simple and achievable.

As you practice your new eating and exercise skills, they will become habits. These new habits will change your life for the better.

As you try to eat better, you will have some challenges. We will discuss some of those challenges and how to meet them in the next steps.

Step 6
Provide Ongoing Motivation

As you implement your plan, obstacles and challenges will begin to surface. Daily motivation becomes critical to your success. What inspires you? Who inspires you? Do you know any inspirational quotes, stories, or sayings that will encourage you to stick with your plan and not give up?

Your own story acts as the core motivation for your weight loss program. It contains your 'motivational whys' and should be reviewed often to avoid discouragement and setbacks. Using the inspirational thoughts and success stories of others can also help you stay motivated and on track. You should think about your own story and add to it often.

How do you stay motivated after hitting a plateau or experiencing a setback? A plateau occurs when you think you're doing all the right things but you're not losing weight.

Setbacks occur when circumstances change and you don't achieve your weekly goals. How do you stay motivated and get back 'on it'? Staying motivated when you get discouraged or experience a setback is very important to your ultimate weight loss success.

Realize that you cannot avoid setbacks and plateaus. They will happen. However, you can choose how you will respond.

Think about an airplane flight. How much planning is done before the plane takes off? What kind of calculations have to be done to make sure that the plane has enough fuel for the flight? After all the planning and the plane is fueled, do the pilots check and make sure there is enough fuel for the flight or do they just take off? Is there only enough fuel for the takeoff? What happens if there is only enough fuel for half the journey? Is there a way to refuel? Is there an airport nearby where the plane can land and refuel? Is it possible that an unexpected storm comes up and forces the plane to land? Without fuel and good planning, a plane could never get off the ground, fly, or reach a destination.

Motivation is the fuel that will get you into the air, stay on your desired course and reach your destination in spite of discouragement and setbacks. Making sure that an airplane has enough fuel is critical to a successful flight. Planning and making sure that you have enough ongoing motivation is critical to your weight loss plan.

I memorized the following poems and review them daily, especially when I am tempted to stray from my weight loss plan:

There can be no fullness of life where there is slavery.
The man who is subject to his appetite is the most abject slave.
The man who can rule his passions is greater than a king.

Author Unknown

Stick to your task, 'til it sticks to you
Beginners are many, enders are few
Honor, power, peace, and praise
Will come in time to the one who stays.

Stick to your task, 'til it sticks to you
Bend at it, sweat at it, smile at it too
For out of the bend and the sweat and the smile
Will come life's victories after awhile.

Author Unknown

Here are a few other examples of inspiring
stories and quotes:

Sew a thought
Reap an act

Sew an act
Reap a habit

Sew a habit
Reap a character

Sew a character
Reap a destiny

Author Unknown

In World War Two, during the battle for
England, when England for a time stood
virtually alone against German aggression,
Germany was pounding London with incessant
bombing. There was the constant threat of
invasion and many were killed. Winston
Churchill inspired his people to continue
resisting with these words: "We shall defend
our island, whatever the cost may be, we shall
fight on the beaches, we shall fight on the
landing grounds, we shall fight in the fields and
in the streets, we shall fight in the hills; we shall
never surrender." His words and leadership

inspired a nation to stay the course and not give up.

Were there setbacks? Did England lose some battles on the road to victory? Where would the world be today if England had given up and surrendered? Winston Churchill understood the importance of developing a successful mindset for himself and his people. He also said, "Success is going from failure to failure without a loss of enthusiasm." The key is never giving up or giving in and being enthusiastic even in the face of adversity.

In the early 1950's, Harland Sanders, known as Colonel Sanders, owned a gas station in Kentucky. He sold gas and served meals to hungry travelers. His meals included his celebrated chicken, made from a recipe that he had perfected over a twenty year period. When a state highway was built that bypassed his store in Corbin, Kentucky, his business dried up and he was left only with his social security check as income. He decided to sell the rights to his chicken for a small piece of the profit on each sale. He travelled from one restaurant to another trying to convince them to pay him to use his recipe. He spoke to over 900 restaurant owners before meeting with Pete Harman, of Salt Lake City, who took the Colonel up on his offer. Pete Harman worked closely with the

Colonel in developing the franchise until
Colonel Sanders sold the franchise in 1964 for
$2,000,000. He continued as a spokesman for
the franchise until his death in 1980.

This quote sums up his life and philosophy: "I
made a resolve then that I was going to amount
to something if I could, and no hours, nor
amount of labor, nor amount of money would
deter me from giving the best that there was in
me. And I have done that ever since, and I win
by it. I know."

Ongoing motivation can be as simple as
reviewing your own story, reminding yourself
why you want to lose weight, being familiar
with the success stories of others, and
memorizing a few simple poems. Mix and
match these techniques as your circumstances
and needs require.

If you choose, you can read the biographies of
people who overcame incredible odds to
become successful, they are all around us.
Learn about some of the following people and
how they became successful; Helen Keller,
George Washington, Ben Franklin, Madame
Curie, Thomas Edison, Henry Ford, Abraham
Lincoln, and Mother Teresa. There are many
great stories about men and women who faced

adversity and achieved their goals. Choose a few of their stories and learn about them. Use their stories and some of their quotes to stay motivated and keep on track.

If you spend time reading about the success of others, write summaries of what impressed you most about their determination, hard work, and persistence that you can review and use for your own motivation.

Why not in our own spheres, add our names to the list of great people. Not that we need to rise to obtain the world's recognition for our accomplishments, but simply that we have made our homes and communities better places to live? Can losing a few pounds do this? I don't know, but you'll feel better, and you'll have more self-esteem. Could you change the world? If you succeed, you've changed yours.

Sharing your success, experience, and what you've learned with others is another way to find encouragement and support. One way to do this is to find a workout partner who has the same concerns and interests as you.

Remembering your successful experiences when the going gets tough or you have a setback can also provide much needed motivation.

Summing It Up

Spend a few minutes each day remembering why you want to lose weight and what your plan is for the day. Review inspirational poems and stories that inspire you and will help you stay 'on it.' You may consider working together with someone who has similar aspirations and goals.

At the end of the day, think about the commitments and the goals you achieved and feel good about them. Take a minute and note your success in your workbook.

Step 7
Interpret Your Results and Adjust Accordingly

Remember that you can get fat again if you go back to your old eating and exercise habits.

During flight, pilots continually check their instruments, making sure their plane is still on course and moving toward its destination. Likewise it's important for you to continue to review your goals and make sure you are achieving the results you want.

Interpreting your results means that on a regular basis (daily or weekly), you are evaluating your progress to determine if a course correction is needed.

In this phase of developing a successful mindset, your plan is fully implemented and you're beginning to see results. You feel better and you're beginning to lose those unwanted pounds. But you have experienced some minor setbacks or you foresee some challenges ahead. Thanksgiving is coming. You've been invited out to eat with some friends. A vacation is coming up. Don't worry. By doing the **5-Minute Mindsetting** steps daily, even if you experience a minor or major setback, you'll be prepared for most challenges and will be able to get back 'on it.' This is the key. You can only fail if you don't get back 'on it.'

Don't be afraid to adjust either your goals or your plan in order to get the results that you want. Determination and persistence will win the day. Try again tomorrow.

You will find that as you begin to implement your plan, things happen. Life in particular has this quality of putting up obstacles that makes writing your new story challenging and difficult. The price of success is higher than anticipated. Someone you admire criticizes your efforts, you become ill, or your employment changes. Whatever it is; life happens and circumstances change.

When I first set my weight loss goals, I really didn't think about how I would feel when Thanksgiving and Christmas rolled around. Like most families, eating is a big event around Thanksgiving and this particular year we were planning to be in Hawaii over the Christmas holiday. I had already lost a lot of weight by Thanksgiving. I could easily have chosen to allow myself some slack. Instead, I chose to stick with my plan and eat within my chosen healthy food groups. Although I allowed myself to eat a little more over Thanksgiving and Christmas, I still continued to lose weight. I was 'on it.'

If you see that a course adjustment is needed, don't try to change too many habits at once. Developing the **5-Minute Mindset** is a process. You will learn as you go. Continue down the path and you will find the resources and help you need as you adjust and change your habits.

Deciding when and what course corrections are needed, requires the ability to evaluate your progress. As you decide on needed course corrections, asking yourself the right questions is very important. Are you learning how to ask yourself the right questions? Here are a few examples: Why have I stopped losing weight? What am I eating that is unhealthy? What foods can I replace them with? What is a healthy amount of fat in a diet? How much should I increase my exercise time every day? Am I losing weight at a healthy rate? Am I achieving my weekly and monthly weight loss goals?

As you evaluate your progress, you may find ways to improve your plan or recognize the need to adjust your weight loss rate.

After implementing my plan, I began losing weight too fast. By too fast, I mean 4 to 5 lbs in two to three days. Research indicates losing weight that fast is unhealthy. I wanted to lose weight at a nice steady pace and keep the weight off for good. So I adjusted my eating in such a way as to slow down the weight loss to a healthier pace. I kept eating plenty of low fat foods, fruits and vegetables, but I ate more of them. I would also allow myself to eat low fat sweets such as low fat cookies, candy and ice cream. There are a number of companies that make good tasting low fat ice cream, cookies, candies, and other products.

After my weight was about the same for a period of time, I would go back to eating smaller portions. In this way I maintained a healthy weight loss rate. It would take awhile before I started getting the results I wanted, losing 2-3 pounds per week.

Having the proper mindset in place from the beginning was critical for me as I evaluated my progress. I made decisions about how much weight to lose in a month and how I was going to eat during a vacation or other event.

Even with the right mindset, you will have unexpected challenges to face. I was involved in a car accident that resulted in some back and neck issues for me. My weight loss program suddenly needed help. I couldn't exercise as much and was in pain all the time. I wanted to eat more. Most of you know what it is like when you don't feel well. In spite of this setback, I was able to keep off most of the weight that I had lost. My mindset and new set of eating habits made this possible. I reviewed my story, my plan and motivations. This encouraged me not to give up but to stick with it. As I began to improve, I was able to get back on track with my weight loss program and began losing weight again.

If you have an unexpected circumstance in your life that takes you off your plan for a time, just remember you can get back 'on it' quickly by repeating steps 1-9. You've already done the steps once; they should fall into place for you faster the next time. Review your story and remind yourself about why you wanted to lose weight. Review your inspirational thoughts or memorize a new one. Maybe stronger motives are needed. Maybe your weight loss goals are too aggressive. Set new monthly weight loss goals. Evaluate your plan and decide what needs to be adjusted if anything. When something unexpected happens feel free to adjust your plans and your goals but keep the ultimate destination in mind. During this evaluation process, you'll get ideas of habits you need to change to accomplish your goals. Don't quit! Today's a new day and success is just around the corner.

You may feel that you do not have control of your own destiny, but you do. You decide what you think about. You decide how you will respond to any challenge.

When Christopher Reeve fell off a horse and became a quadriplegic, he had to change the course and direction of his life and develop a new set of habits and a new lifestyle. With amazing determination and courage, and with the help of his wife and others, he created a new life for himself.

If you have a setback, be sure to re-read your story in your workbook. Look at the resources you have that might help. As you review your successes and failures, focus on the successes and re-commit to the habits that brought you success. Recommitting to successful habits will lead to a brighter and happier future.

You will find that during your weight loss journey, you will need to make occasional course adjustments. Stick with your general plan. After getting back 'on it,' it would sometimes take me two to three days or longer before I began to lose weight again. It was at times like these that having the proper mindset and knowing how to keep it were very important.

When you experience a setback or get discouraged, decide to stay with your overall plan and don't quit. During a course adjustment, if you get discouraged, go back to your story and write about what is going on in your workbook, decide how you are going to improve. Adjust your goals, re-commit to your new eating and exercise habits. Keep it simple and stay with it!!! You can do it.

If your weight loss program includes weightlifting, be aware that toned muscle is heavier than un-toned muscle. Initially, you may gain weight until you build your muscles up and your new eating habits begin to take effect. As mentioned previously, I have always enjoyed lifting weights. My muscles were quite well toned, but I still wasn't able to lose weight. After going through the mindsetting process, I realized that I needed to change my bad eating habits. This was a major course correction for me. I re-did my eating plan and committed to the change. This helped me keep my commitments through Thanksgiving and Christmas and lose 73 pounds in the process. Were there days when I allowed myself to eat a little more? Yes, but I ate foods that were allowed within my weight loss plan.

Don't worry about the daily weight fluctuations. I weigh myself Monday through Saturday at the gym. Some days my weight goes up a pound then it drops two. It takes time before you will begin to see some weight loss from your plan. Don't panic if you don't see immediate results. Take an honest look at your plan and decide if something has to change or if you will stay the course.

Learning how to lose weight takes time. As I engaged in the **5-Minute Mindsetting** process, it wasn't hard to see what eating habits I needed to change. Even now as I go to different restaurants and places to eat, I remember the general rules that are in place and order accordingly.

Once you have the right mindset, eating right gets easier. Recently I decided to go out and eat anything I wanted. Once I got to the restaurant, I ordered my usual broccoli, barbecued chicken, plain baked potato and water. I planned to cheat but couldn't, and found myself satisfied and full with the good foods that help me lose and maintain my weight.

In Summary

Avoid falling back into your old eating and
exercise habits by spending a few minutes every
day reviewing your weight loss plan. Think
about your goals for the day and remember why
you want to lose weight.

Are you 'on it' today or do you need a breather?
Make course adjustments, if needed, to better fit
your current circumstances. Never lose sight of
your overall goal. If you are struggling with
motivation, talk with a friend or your workout
partner. You can also stay motivated by
reviewing your story and remembering how
important new eating and exercise habits are to
you. Write these ideas in your workbook.

If you are involved in the process, you've seen
some success. If you aren't seeing the success
you want, then check each of the previous steps
and ask yourself how you can engage in these
steps more proactively? The more involved you
become in the **5-Minute Mindsetting** process,
the better you will understand it and the more
success you will have.

Step 8
Celebrate Your Success

Celebrating your success along the way is an important feature of the **5-Minute Mindsetting** process. During each phase it's important to celebrate your successes no matter how small they may be. When you lose that first pound, celebrate it. The sooner you begin to have some success and celebrate it, the more likely you are to go on and complete the next step of the process.

You should plan little ways to celebrate your successes. Celebrating a success can be as simple as writing in your workbook, "I did it," or allowing yourself to eat a little more of your favorite low fat treat. You might even plan a vacation or buy better fitting clothes for reaching a major weight loss goal.

Part of celebrating your success is sharing what you've learned and accomplished with others.

Nothing is more satisfying than seeing a friend or acquaintance pick up a few ideas that can make such a difference in their lives and see them move down the path of successful weight loss.

Watching others succeed is very motivating. My brother and sister-in-law began applying the principles in this book and began to see immediate results.

Experiencing the joy of others' success is a very satisfying way to celebrate your own success.

Celebrate every success as part of your **5-Minute Mindsetting** journey.

Step 9
Arrive at Your Destination

As a plane comes in for a landing, pilots check the landing gear instruments and other systems to make sure all is ready for landing. Landing is another dangerous phase for the pilots. Anything can happen and different circumstances can make the landing very dangerous. If you are well prepared and trained, landing can be the best part of any flight.

After achieving your weight loss goals, it is important to maintain the right mindset and your new eating and exercise habits.

You are eating healthier foods and exercising regularly. You have stayed motivated and are excited to move on to other goals. Be careful. Don't forget what you have learned about eating and exercising. Avoid falling back into bad habits and continue to monitor and evaluate where you are in regards to your weight.

As your plane taxis to the terminal, remember how much you've changed and enjoy it. You've gained self esteem, inner strength, and formed new habits. You are greater than a king or queen.

By spending just five minutes a day, you can maintain a powerful mindset. By reviewing your 'whys', goals, and plans just a few minutes a day, you'll keep those great eating and exercise habits in place and maintain that ideal weight.

Remember to keep your new weight loss mindset intact.

You may choose to go on to other goals and master other talents and skills that you have.

The **5-Minute Mindsetting** process will be equally valuable in these areas.

Good luck with your ongoing **5-Minute Mindsetting** adventures.

Acknowledgements

I'd like to thank the following people:

My wife and family for their encouragement and ideas.

My brother Rick, for helping me develop the steps of **The 5-Minute Mindset.**

Tonya Roberts, for her input and help in editing the book.

Travis Kelly, for visually capturing my story with his amazing cartoons.

About the Author

Bob is a Real Estate Broker by profession. He has worked in the Real Estate industry since 1985.

Over the years he has trained hundreds of agents in the art of successful sales and marketing.

From 1988 to 2008 he served as president of Rocky Mountain Mortgage Inc., developing a very successful program that generated thousands of loans in over eight states.

What he learned over these years as a successful businessman certainly qualifies him as a man who understands the importance of having the right mindset in achieving success.

Now he is applying the same mindsetting principles to weight loss and sharing his success with others through **The 5-Minute Mindset for Weight Loss.**

www.ingramcontent.com/pod-product-compliance
Lightning Source LLC
Chambersburg PA
CBHW060909280326
41934CB00007B/1243